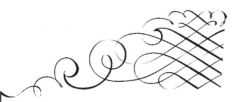

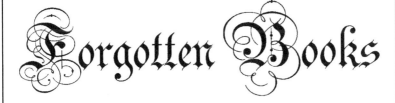
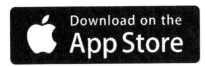
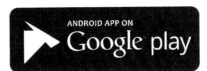

ISBN 978-1-332-11687-4
PIBN 10286903

This book is a reproduction of an important historical work. Forgotten Books uses state-of-the-art technology to digitally reconstruct the work, preserving the original format whilst repairing imperfections present in the aged copy. In rare cases, an imperfection in the original, such as a blemish or missing page, may be replicated in our edition. We do, however, repair the vast majority of imperfections successfully; any imperfections that remain are intentionally left to preserve the state of such historical works.

1 MONTH OF
FREE
READING

at

www.ForgottenBooks.com

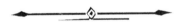

By purchasing this book you are eligible for one month membership to ForgottenBooks.com, giving you unlimited access to our entire collection of over 700,000 titles via our web site and mobile apps.

To claim your free month visit:

www.forgottenbooks.com/free286903

LETTER

ON

CORPULENCE,

Addressed to the Public

By WILLIAM BANTING.

REPRINTED FROM THE THIRD LONDON EDITION.

WITH A REVIEW OF THE WORK FROM
BLACKWOOD'S MAGAZINE,

AND AN ARTICLE ON

CORPULENCY & LEANNESS

FROM HARPER'S WEEKLY.

SAN FRANCISCO:
PUBLISHED BY A. ROMAN & CO.
417 & 419 MONTGOMERY STREET.

1865.

This letter is respectfully dedicated to the Public simply and entirely from an earnest desire to confer a a benefit on my fellow creatures.

W. B.

BANTING ON CORPULENCE.

Of all the parasites that affect humanity, I do not know of, nor can I imagine, any more distressing than that of Obesity, and, having just emerged from a very long probation in this affliction, I am desirous of circulating my humble knowledge and experience for the benefit of my fellow man, with an earnest hope it may lead to the same comfort and happiness I now feel under the extraordinary change—which might almost be termed miraculous, had it not been accomplished by the most simple common-sense means.

Obesity seems to me very little understood or properly appreciated by the faculty and the public generally, or the former would long ere this have hit upon the cause for so lamentable a disease, and applied effective remedies, whilst the latter would have spared their injudicious indulgence in remarks and sneers, frequently painful in society, and which, even on the strongest mind, have an unhappy tendency; but I sincerely trust this humble effort at exposition may lead to a more perfect ventilation of the subject and a better feeling for the afflicted.

It would afford me infinite pleasure and satisfaction to name the author of my redemption from the calamity, as he is the only one that I have been able to find (and my search has not been sparing) who seems

2A

thoroughly up in the question; but such publicity might be construed improperly, and I have, therefore, only to offer my personal experience as the stepping-stone to public investigation, and to proceed with my narrative of facts, earnestly hoping the reader will patiently peruse and thoughtfully consider it, with forbearance for any fault of style or diction, and for any seeming presumption in publishing it.

I have felt some difficulty in deciding on the proper and best course of action. At one time I thought the Editor of the *Lancet* would kindly publish a letter from me on the subject, but further reflection led me to doubt whether an insignificant individual would be noticed without some special introduction. In the April number of the *Cornhill Magazine* I read with much interest an article on the subject—defining tolerably well the effects, but offering no tangible remedy, or even positive solution of the problem—"What is the cause of Obesity?" I was pleased with the article as a whole, but objected to some portions, and had prepared a letter to the Editor of that Magazine, offer-ing my experience on the subject; but again it struck me that an unknown individual like myself would have but little prospect of notice; so I finally resolved to publish and circulate this Pamphlet, with no other reason, motive, or expectation than an earnest desire to help those who happen to be afflicted as I was, for that corpulence is remediable I am well convinced, and shall be delighted if I can induce others to think so. The object I have in view impels me to enter into minute particulars, as well as general observations, and to revert to bygone years, in order to show that I have spared no pains nor expense to accomplish the great end of stopping and curing obesity.

I am now nearly 66 years of age, about 5 feet 5 inches in stature, and in August last (1862), weighed 202 lbs., which I think it right to name, because the article in the *Cornhill Magazine* presumes that a certain stature and age should bear ordinarily a certain weight, and I am quite of that opinion. I now weigh 167 lbs., showing a diminution of something like 1lb. per week since August, and having now very nearly attained the happy medium, I have perfect confidence that a few more weeks will fully accomplish the object for which I have labored for the last thirty years, in vain, until it pleased Almighty Providence to direct me into the right and proper channel — the "tramway," so to speak—of happy, comfortable existence

Few men have led a more active life—bodily or mentally—from a constitutional anxiety for regularity, precision, and order, during fifty years' business career, from which I have now retired, so that my corpulence and subsequent obesity was not through neglect of necessary bodily activity, nor from excessive eating, drinking, or self-indulgence of any kind, except that I partook of the simple aliments of bread, milk, butter, beer, sugar, and potatoes more freely than my aged nature required, and hence, as I believe, the generation of the parasite, detrimental to comfort. if not really to health.

I will not presume to descant on the bodily structural tissues, so fully canvassed in the *Cornhill Magazine*, nor how they are supported and renovated, having no mind or power to enter into those questions, which properly belong to the wise heads of the faculty. None of my family on the side of either parent had any tendency to corpulence, and from my earliest years I had an inexpressible dread of such a calamity, so, when I

was between tiirty and forty years of age, finding a
tendency to it creeping upon me, I consulted an eminent surgeon, now long deceased—a kind personal
friend—who recommended increased bodily exertion
before my ordinary daily labors began, and tiougit
rowing an excellent plan. I iad tie command of a
good, ieavy, safe boat, lived near tie river, and
adopted it for a couple of iours in tie early morning.
It is true I gained muscular vigor, but witi it a
prodigious appetite, wiici I was compelled to indulge,
and consequently increased in weigit, until my kind
old friend advised me to forsake tie exercise.

He soon afterwards died, and, as tie tendency to
corpulence remained, I consulted otier iigi ortiodox
autiorities (*never any inferior adviser*), but all in vain.
I iave tried sea air and batiing in various localities,
witi muci walking exercise ; taken gallons of piysic
and liquor potassæ, advisedly and abundantly ; riding
on iorseback ; tie waters and climate of Leamington
many times, as well as tiose of Cielteniam and Har-
rogate frequently ; iave lived upon sixpence a day, so
to speak, and earned it, if bodily labor may be so
construed ; and iave spared no trouble nor expense in
consultations witi tie best autiorities in tie land,
giving eaci and all a fair time for experiment, witiout
any permanent remedy, as tie evil still gradually
increased.

I am under obligations to most of tiose advisers for
tie pains and interest tiey took in my case ; but only
to one for an effectual remedy.

Wien a corpulent man eats, drinks, and sleeps
well, ias no pain to complain of, and no particular
organic disease, tie judgment of able men seems paral
yzed—for I iave been generally informed tiat corpu-

lence is one of the natural results of increasing years ; indeed, one of the ablest authorities as a physician in the land told me he had gained 1 lb. in weight every year since he attained manhood, and was not surprised at my condition, but advised more bodily exercise— vapor-baths and shampooing, in addition to the medicine given. Yet the evil still increased, and, like the parasite of barnacles on a ship, if it did not destroy the structure, it obstructed its fair, comfortable progress in the path of life.

I have been in dock, perhaps twenty times in as many years, for the reduction of this disease, and with little good effect—none lasting. Any one so afflicted is often subject to public remark, and though in conscience he may care little about it, I am confident no man laboring under obesity can be quite insensible to the sneers and remarks of the cruel and injudicious in public assemblies, public vehicles or the ordinary street traffic ; nor to the annoyance of finding no adequate space in a public assembly if he should seek amusement or need refreshment, and therefore he naturally keeps away as much as possible from places where he is likely to be made the object of the taunts and remarks of others. I am as regardless of public remark as most men, but I have felt these difficulties and therefore avoided such circumscribed accommodation and notice, and by that means have been deprived of many advantages to health and comfort.

Although no very great size or weight, still I could not stoop to tie my shoe, so to speak, nor attend to the little offices humanity requires, without considerable pain and difficulty, which only the corpulent can understand ; I have been compelled to go down stairs slowly backwards, to save the jar of increased weight upon the ancle and knee-joints, and been obliged to puff and blow with every slight exertion, particularly that of going up stairs. I have spared no pains to remedy this by low living (*moderation and light food* was generally prescribed, but I had no direct bill of fare to know what was really intended), and that, consequently, brought the system into a low, impoverished state, without decreasing corpulence, caused many obnoxious boils to appear, and two rather formidable carbuncles, for which I was ably operated upon and *fed into increased obesity.*

At this juncture (about three years back) Turkish baths became the fashion, and I was advised to adopt them as a remedy. With the first few I found immense benefit in power and elasticity for walking exercise ; so, believing I had found the "philosopher's stone," pursued them three times a week till I had taken fifty, then less frequently (as I began to fancy, with some reason, that so many weakened my constitution) till I had taken ninety, but never succeeded in losing more than 6 lbs. weight during the whole course, and I gave up the plan as worthless ; though I have full belief in their cleansing properties, and their value in colds, rheumatism, and many other ailments.

I then fancied increasing obesity materially affected a slight umbilical rupture, if it did not cause it, and that another bodily ailment to which I had been subject was also augmented. This led me to other medical advisers, to whom I am also indebted for much kind consideration, though, unfortunately, they failed in relieving me. At last finding my sight failing and my hearing greatly impaired, I consulted in August last an eminent aural surgeon, who made light of the case, looked into my ears, sponged them internally,

and blistered the outside, without the slightest benefit,
neither inquiring into any of my bodily ailments, which
he probably thought unnecessary, nor affording me
even time to name them.

I was not at all satisfied, but on the contrary, was
in a worse plight than when I went to him ; however,
he soon after left town for his annual holiday, which
proved the greatest possible blessing to me, because it
compelled me to seek other assistance, and, happily, I
found the right man, who unhesitatingly said he be
lieved my ailments were caused principally by corpulence, and prescribed a certain diet,—no medicine,
beyond a morning cordial as a corrective, — with
immense effect and advantage both to my hearing and
the decrease of my corpulency.

For the sake of argument and illustration I will pre
sume that certain articles of ordinary diet, however beneficial in youth, are prejudicial in advanced life, like
beans to a horse, whose common ordinary food is hay
and corn. It may be useful food occasionally, under
peculiar circumstances, but detrimental as a constancy.
I will, therefore, adopt the analogy, and call such food
human beans. The items from which I was advised
to abstain as much as possible were :—Bread, butter,
milk, sugar, beer and potatoes, which had been the
main (and I thought innocent) elements of my existence, or, at all events, they had for many years been
adopted freely.

These said my excellent adviser, contain starch
and saccharine matter, tending to create fat, and should
be avoided altogether. At the first blush it seemed
to me that I had little left to live upon, but my kind
friend soon showed me there was ample, and I was
only too happy to give the plan a fair trial, and within

a very few days, found immense benefit from it.   It
may better elucidate the dietary plan if I describe
generally wiat I iave sanction to take, and tiat man
must be an extraordinary person wio would desire a
better table ·—

> For breakfast, I take four or five ounces of beef,
> mutton, kidneys, broiled fisi, bacon, or cold
> meat of any kind except pork ; a large cup of
> tea (witiout milk or sugar), a little biscuit, or
> one ounce of dry toast.
>
> For dinner, Five or six ounces of any fish except
> salmon, any meat except pork, any vegetable
> except potato, one ounce of dry toast, fruit out
> of a pudding, any kind of poultry or game,
> and two or tiree glasses of good claret, sierry,
> or Madeira—Ciampagne, Port and Beer for
> bidden.
>
> For tea, two or tiree ounces of fruit, a rusk or
> two, and a cup of tea witiout milk or sugar.
>
> For supper, Tiree or four ounces of meat or fisi
> similar·to dinner, with a glass or two of claret.
>
> For nigitcap, if required, a tumbler of grog—
> (gin, wiisky or brandy, witiout sugar)—or a
> glass or two of claret or sierry.

Tiis plan leads to an excellent nigit's rest, with
from six to eigit iours' sound sleep.   Tie dry toast
or rusk may iave a table spoonful of spirit to soften
it, wiici will prove acceptable.   Periaps I did not
wiolly escape starciy or sacciarine matter, but scru
pulously avoided tiose beans, suci as milk, sugar,
beer, butter, &c., wiici were known to contain tiem.

On rising in tie morning I take a table spoonful
of a special corrective cordial, wiici may be called tie

Balm of Life, in a wine-glass of water, a most grateful draught, as it seems to carry away all the dregs left in the stomach after digestion, but is not aperient; then I take about 5 or 6 ounces solid and 8 of liquid for breakfast; 8 ounces of solid and 8 of liquid for dinner; 3 ounces of solid and 8 of liquid for tea; 4 ounces of solid and 6 of liquid for supper, and the grog afterwards, if I please. I am not, however, strictly limited to any quantity at either meal, so that the nature of the food is rigidly adhered to.

Experience has taught me to believe that these human beans are the most insidious enemies man, with a tendency to corpulence in advanced life, can possess, though eminently friendly to youth. He may very prudently mount guard against such an enemy if he is not a fool to himself; and I fervently hope this truthful unvarnished tale may lead him to make a trial of my plan, which I sincerely recommend to public notice,—not with any ambitious motive, but in sincere good faith to help my fellow-creatures to obtain the marvellous blessings I have found within the short period of a few months.

I do not recommend every corpulent man to rush headlong into such a change of diet, (*certainly not*), but to act advisedly and after full consultation with a physician.

My former dietary table was bread and milk for breakfast, or a pint of tea with plenty of milk and sugar, and buttered toast; meat, beer, much bread (of which I was always very fond) and pastry for dinner, the meal of tea similar to that of breakfast, and generally a fruit tart or bread and milk for supper. I had little comfort and far less sound sleep.

It certainly appears to me that my present dietary

table is far superior to the former—more luxurious
and liberal, independent of its blessed effect—but
when it is proved to be more healthful, comparisons
are simply ridiculous, and I can hardly imagine any
man, even in sound health, would choose the former,
even if it were not an enemy ; but, when it is shown
to be, as in my case, inimical both to health and comfort, I can hardly conceive there is any man who
would not willingly avoid it.   I can conscientiously
assert I never lived so well as under the new plan of
dietary, which I should have formerly thought a dangerous extravagant trespass upon health ; I am very
much better, bodily and mentally, and pleased to believe that I hold the reins of health and comfort in
my own hands, and, though at sixty-five years of age,
I cannot expect to remain free from some coming
natural infirmity that all flesh is heir to, I cannot at
the present time complain of one. It is simply miraculous, and I am thankful to Almighty Providence for
directing me, through an extraordinary change, to the
care of a man who could work such a chance in so
short a time.

On ! that the faculty would look deeper into and
make themselves better acquainted with the crying evil
of obesity—that dreadful tormenting parasite on health
and comfort.   Their fellow men might not descend into
early premature graves, as I believe many do, from
what is termed apoplexy, and certainly would not,
during their sojourn on earth, endure so much bodily
and consequently mental infirmity.

Corpulence, though giving no actual pain, as it
appears to me, must naturally press with undue vio-
lence upon the bodily viscera, driving one part upon
another, and stopping the free action of all. I am

sure it did in my particular case, and the result of my experience is briefly as follows

I have not felt so well as now for the last twenty years.

Have suffered no inconvenience whatever in the probational remedy.

Am reduced many inches in bulk, and 35lbs. in weight in thirty-eight weeks.

Come down stairs forward naturally with perfect ease.

Go up stairs and take ordinary exercise freely, without the slightest inconvenience.

Can perform every necessary office for myself.

The umbilical rupture is greatly ameliorated, and gives me no anxiety.

My sight is restored—my hearing improved.

My other bodily ailments are ameliorated ; indeed, almost past into matter of history.

I have placed a thank-offering of £50 in the hands of my kind medical adviser for distribution amongst his favorite hospitals, after gladly paying his usual fees, and still remain under overwhelming obligations for his care and attention, which I can never hope to repay. Most thankful to Almighty Providence for mercies received, and determined to press the case into public notice as a token of gratitude.

I have the pleasure to afford, in conclusion, a satisfactory confirmation of my report, in stating that a corpulent friend of mine, who, like myself, is possessed of a generally sound constitution, was labouring under frequent palpitations of the heart and sensations of fainting, was, at my instigation, induced to place himself in the hands of my medical adviser, with the same gradual beneficial results. He is at present under the same ordeal, and in eight weeks has profited even more largely tian I did in tiat siort period ; ie ias lost tie palpitations, and is becoming, so to speak, a new made man—tiankful to me for advising, and grateful to tie eminent counsellor to wiom I referred iim—and ie looks forward witi good iope to a perfect cure.

I am fully persuaded that iundreds, if not tiousands, of our fellow men migit profit equally by a similar course ; but, constitutions not being all alike, a different course of treatment may be advisable for tie removal of so tormenting an affliction.

My kind and valued medical adviser is not a doctor for obesity, but stands on tie pinnacle of fame in tie treatment of anotier malady, wiici, as ie well knows, is frequently induced by tie disease of wiici I am speaking, and I most sincerely trust most of my corpulent friends (and tiere are tiousands of corpulent people wiom I dare not so rank) may be led into my tramroad. To any suci I am prepared to offer tie furtier key of knowledge by naming tie man. It migit seem invidious to do so now, but I siall only be too iappy, if applied to by letter in good faiti, or if any doubt siould exist as to tie correctness of tiis statement.

WILLIAM BANTING, Sen.,

Late of No. 27 *St. James's Street, Piccadilly,*

Now of No. 4, *The Terrace, Kensington.*

May, 1863.

ADDENDA.

HAVING exhausted the first Edition (1,000 copies) of the foregoing Pamphlet; and a period of one year having elapsed since commencing the admirable course of diet which has led to such inestimably beneficial results, and, "as I expected, and desired," having quite succeeded in attaining the happy medium of weight and bulk I had so long ineffectually sought, *which appears necessary to health at my age and stature* —I feel impelled by a sense of public duty, to offer the result of my experience in a second Edition. It has been suggested that I should have sold the Pamphlet, devoting any profit to Charity as more agreeable and useful; and I had intended to adopt such a course, but on reflection feared my motives might be mistaken; I, therefore, respectfully present this (like the first Edition) to the Public gratuitously, earnestly hoping the subject may be taken up by medical men and thoroughly ventilated.

It may (and I hope will) be, as satisfactory to the public to hear, as it is for me to state, that the first Edition has been attended with very comforting results to other sufferers from Corpulence, as the remedial system therein described was to me under that terrible disease, which was my main object in publishing my convictions on the subject. It has moreover attained a success, produced flattering compliments, and an amount of attention I could hardly have imagined possible. The pleasure and satisfaction this has afforded me, is ample compensation for tie trouble and expense I 1ave incurred, and I most sincerely trust, "as I verily believe," tiis second Edition will be accompanied by similar satisfactory results from a more extensive circulation. If so, it will inspirit me to circulate furtier Editions, w1ilst a corpulent person exists, requiring, as I t1ink, tiis system of diet, or so·long as my motives cannot be mistaken, and are t1ankfully appreciated.

My weigit is reduced 46℔s., and as tie *very gradual reductions* w1ic1 I am able to s1ow may be, interesting to many, I 1ave great pleasure in stating t1em, believing t1ey serve to demonstrate furt1er t1e merit of t1e system pursued.

My weigit on 26th August, 1862, was 202℔s.

		℔s.		℔s.
On 7th September, it was		200,	1aving lost	2
27th "	"	197	"	3 more
19t1 October	"	193	"	4 "
9th November	"	190	"	3 "
3rd December	"	187	"	3 "
24th "		184	"	3 "
14t1 Jan., 1863	"	182	"	2 "
4th February	"	180	"	2 "
25th	"	178	"	2 "
18t1 Marc1	··	176	"	2 "
8t1 April	··	173	"	3 "
29th "		170	"	3 "
20th May	"	167	"	3 "
10th June		164	"	3 "
1st July		161	"	3 "
22nd "		159	"	2 "
12t1 August	"	157	"	2 "
26th "		156	"	1 "
12t1 September	"	156	"	0 "

Total loss of weigit............ 46℔s.

My girth is . reduced round the waist, in tailor phraseology, 12¼ inches, which extent was hardly conceivable even by my own friends, or my respected medical adviser, until I put on my former clothing, over what I now wear, which was a thoroughly convincing proof of the remarkable change. These important desiderata have been attained by the most easy and comfortable means, with but little medicine, and almost entirely by a system of diet, that formerly I should have thought dangerously generous. I am told by all who know me that my personal appearance is greatly improved, and that I seem to bear the stamp of good health; this may be a matter of opinion or friendly remark, but I can honestly assert that I feel restored in health, " bodily and mentally," appear to have more muscular power and vigour, eat and drink with a good appetite, and sleep well. All symptoms of acidity, indigestion, and heartburn, (with which I was frequently tormented) have vanished. I have left off using boot hooks, and other such aids which were indispensible, but being now able to stoop with ease and freedom, are unnecessary. I have lost the feeling of *occasional faintness*, and what I think a remarkable blessing and comfort is that I have been able safely to leave off knee bandages, which I had worn *necessarily* for 20 past years, and given up a truss almost entirely; indeed I believe I might wholly discard it with safety, but am advised to wear it at least occasionally for the present.

Since publishing my Pamphlet, I have felt constrained to send a copy of it to my former medical advisers, and to ascertain their opinions on the subject. They did not dispute or question the propriety of the system, but either dared not venture its practice upon

B

a man of my age, or thought it too great a sacrifice of personal comfort to be generally advised or adopted, and I fancy none of them appeared to feel the fact of the misery of corpulence. One eminent physician, as I before stated, assured me that increasing weight was a necessary result of advancing years; another equally eminent, to whom I had been directed by a very friendly third, who had most kindly but ineffectually failed in a remedy, added to my weight in a few weeks instead of abating the evil. These facts lead me to believe the question is not sufficiently observed or even regarded.

The great charm and comfort of the system is, that its effects are palpable within a week of trial, which creates a natural stimulus to persevere for a few weeks more, when the fact becomes established beyond question.

I only entreat all persons suffering from corpulence to make a fair trial for just one clear month, as I am well convinced they will afterwards pursue a course which yields such extraordinary benefit, till entirely and effectually relieved; and be it remembered, by the sacrifice merely of simple, for the advantage of more generous and comforting food. The simple dietary evidently adds fuel to fire, whereas the superior and liberal seems to extinguish it.

I am delighted to be able to assert that I have proved the great merit and advantage of the system by its result in several other cases, similar to my own, and have full confidence that within the next twelve months I shall know of many more cases restored from the disease of corpulence, for I have received the kindest possible letters from many afflicted strangers and friends, as well as similar personal observations from others whom I have conversed with, and assurances from most of them that they will kindly inform me the result for my own private satisfaction. Many are practicing the diet after consultation with their own medical advisers ; some few have gone to mine, and others are practicing upon their own convictions of the advantages detailed in the Pamphlet, though I recommend all to act advisedly, in case their constitutions should differ. I am, however, so perfectly satisfied of the great unerring benefits of this system of diet, that I shall spare no trouble to circulate my humble experience. The amount and character of my correspondence on the subject has been strange and singular, but most satisfactory to my mind and feelings.

I am now in that happy, comfortable state, that I should not hesitate to indulge in any fancy in regard to diet, but if I did so, should watch the consequences, and not continue any course which might add to weight or bulk and consequent discomfort.

Is not the system suggestive to artists and men of sedentary employment, who cannot spare time for exercise, consequently become corpulent, and clog the little muscular action with a superabundance of fat, thus easily avoided ?

Pure genuine bread may be the staff of life, as it is termed. It is so, particularly in youth, but I feel certain it is more wholesome in advanced life if thoroughly toasted, as I take it. My impression is, that any starchy or saccharine matter tends to the disease of corpulence in advanced life, and whether it be swallowed in that form, or generated in the stomach, that all things tending to these elements should be avoided, of course always under sound medical authority.

WILLIAM BANTING.

CONCLUDING ADDENDA.

It is very satisfactory to me to be able to state, that I remained at the same standard of bulk and weight for several weeks after the 26th August, when I attained the happy natural medium, since which time I have varied in weight from two to three pounds, more or less. I have seldom taken the morning draught since that time, and have frequently indulged my fancy, *experimentally*, in using milk, sugar, butter and potatoes—indeed, I may say, all the forbidden articles, *except beer*, in moderation, with impunity, but always as an exception, not as a rule. This deviation, however, convinces me that I hold the power of maintaining the happy medium in my own hands.

A kind friend has lately furnished me with a tabular statement in regard to weight as proportioned to stature, which, under present circumstances and the new movement, may be interesting and useful to corpulent readers :—

STATURE.			WEIGHT.				
5 feet 1	should be	8 stone	8	or	120 lbs.		
5 " 2	"	9	"	0	"	126	"
5 " 3	"	9	"	7	"	133	"
5 " 4	"	9	"	10	"	136	"
5 " 5	"	10	"	2	"	142	"
5 " 6	"	10	"	5	"	145	"
5 " 7	"	10	"	8	"	148	"
5 " 8	"	11	"	1	"	155	"
5 " 9	"	11	"	8	"	162	"
5 " 10	"	12	"	1	"	169	"
5 " 11	"	12	"	6	"	174	"
6 " 0	"	12	"	10	"	178	"

This tabular statement, taken from a mean average of 2,648 healthy men, was formed and arranged for an Insurance Company, by the late Dr. John Hutchin son. It answered as a pretty good standard, and insurances were regulated upon it. His calculations were made upon the volume of air passing in and out of the lungs, and this was his guide as to how far the various organs of the body were in health, and the lungs in particular. It may be viewed as some sort of probable rule, yet only as an average—some in health weighing more by many pounds than others. It must not be looked upon as infallible, but only as a sort of general reasonable guide to Nature's great and mighty work.

On a general view of the question, I think it may be conceded that a frame of low stature was hardly intended to bear very heavy weight. Judging from this tabular statement I ought to be considerably lighter than I am at present : I shall not, however, covet or aim at such a result, nor, on the other hand, feel alarmed if I decrease a little more in weight and bulk.

I am certainly more sensitive to cold since I have lost the superabundant fat ; but this is remedible by another garment, far more agreeable and satisfactory. Many of my friends have said, "Oh ! you have done well so far, but take care you don't go too far." I fancy such a circumstance, with such a dietary, very unlikely, if not impossible ; but feeling that I have now nearly attained the right standard of bulk and weight proportional to my stature and age (between 10 and 11 stone), I should not hesitate to partake of a fattening dietary occasionally, to preserve that happy standard, if necessary ; indeed, I am allowed to do so by my medical adviser, but I shall always observe a careful watch upon myself to discover the effect, and act accordingly, so that, if I choose to spend a day or two with Dives, so to speak, I must not forget to devote the next to Lazarus.

The remedy may be as old as the hills, as I have since been told, but its application is of very recent date; and it astonishes me that such a light should have remained so long unnoticed and hidden, as not to afford a glimmer to my anxious mind in a search for it during the last twenty years, even in directions where it might have been expected to be known. I would rather presume it is a new light, than that it was purposely hidden, merely because the disease of obesity was not immediately dangerous to existence, nor thought to be worthy of serious consideration. Little do the faculty imagine the misery and bitterness to life through the parasite of corpulence or obesity.

I can now confidently say that *quantity* of diet may be safely left to the natural appetite; and that it is the *quality* only, which is essential to abate and cure corpulence. I stated the quantities of my own dietary, because it was part of a truthful report; but some correspondents have doubted whether it should be more or less in their own cases, a doubt which would be better solved by their own appetite, or medical adviser. I have heard a graphic remark by a corpulent man, which may not be inappropriately stated here, *that big houses were not formed with scanty materials.* This, however, is a poor excuse for self-indulgence in improper food, or for not consulting medical authority.

The approach of corpulence is so gradual that, until it is far advanced, persons rarely become objects of attention. Many may have even congratulated themselves on their comely appearance, and have not sought advice or a remedy for what they did not consider an evil, for an evil I can say most truly it is, when in much excess, to which point it must, in my opinion arrive, unless obviated by proper means.

Many have wished to know (as future readers may) the nature of the morning draught, or where it could be obtained, but believing it would have been highly imprudent on my part to have presumed that what was proper for my constitution was applicable to all indiscriminately, I could only refer them to a medical adviser for any aid beyond the dietary ; assuring them however, it was not a dram but of an alkaline character.

Some, I believe, would willingly submit to even a violent remedy, so that an immediate benefit could be produced ; this is not the object of the treatment, as it cannot but be dangerous, in my humble opinion, to reduce a disease of this nature suddenly ; they are probably then too prone to despair of success, and consider it as unalterably connected with their constitution. Many under this feeling doubtless return to their former habits, encouraged so to act by the ill-judged advice of friends who, I am persuaded (from the correspondence I have had on this most interesting subject) become unthinking accomplices in the destruction of those whom they regard and esteem.

The question of four meals a-day, and the night cap, has been abundantly and amusingly criticized. I ought perhaps to have stated as an excuse for such liberality of diet, that I breakfast between eight and nine o'clock, dine between one and two, take my slight tea meal between five and six, sup at nine, and only take the night-cap when inclination directs. My object in naming it at all was, that, as a part of a whole sys-

tem, it should be known, and to show it is not forbidden to those who are advised that they need such a
luxury ; nor was it injurious in my case. Some have
inquired whether smoking was prohibited. It was
not.

It has also been remarked that such a dietary as
mine was too good and expensive for a poor man, and
that I had wholly lost sight of that class ; but a very
poor corpulent man is not so frequently met with, inasmuch as the poor cannot afford the simple inexpen-
sive means for creating fat ; but when the tendency
does exist in that class, I have no doubt it can be
remedied by abstinence from the forbidden articles,
and a moderate indulgence in such cheap stimulants as
may be recommended by a medical adviser, whom they
have ample chances of consulting gratuitously.

I have a very strong feeling that gout (another
terrible parasite upon humanity) might be greatly
relieved, if not cured entirely, by this proper natural
dietary, and sincerely hope some person so afflicted
may be induced to practice the harmless plan for three
months (as I certainly would if the case were my own)
to prove it ; but not without advice.

My impression from the experiments I have tried
on myself of late is, that saccharine matter is the great
moving cause of fatty corpulence. I know that it produces in my individual case increased weight and a
large amount of flatulence, and believe, that not only
sugar, but all elements tending to create saccharine
matter in the process of digestion, should be avoided.
I apprehend it will be found in bread, butter, milk,
beer, Port wine, and Champagne ; I have not found
starchy matter so troublesome as the saccharine, which
I think, largely increases acidity as well as fat, but,

with ordinary care and observation, people will soon find what food rests easiest in the stomach, and avoid that which does not, during the probationary trial of the proposed dietary. Vegetables and ripe or stewed fruit I have found ample aperients. Failing this, medical advice should be sought.

The word "*parasite*," has been much commented upon, as inappropriate to any but a living creeping thing (of course I use the word in a figurative sense, as a burden to the flesh), but if fat is not an insidious creeping enemy, I do not know what is. .I should have equally applied the word to gout, rheumatism, dropsy, and many other diseases.

Whereas hitherto the appeals to me to know the name of my medical adviser have been very numerous, I may say hundreds, which I have gladly answered, though forming no small item of the expense incurred, and whereas the very extensive circulation expected of the third edition is likely to lead to some thousands of similar applications, I feel bound, in self-defence, to state that the medical gentleman to whom I am so deeply indebted is Mr. Harvey, Soho Square, London, whom I consulted for deafness. In the first and second editions, I thought that to give his name would appear like a puff, which I know he abhors; indeed, I should prefer not to do so now, but cannot, in justice to myself, incur further probable expense (which I fancy inevitable) besides the personal trouble, for which I cannot afford time, and, therefore, feel no hesitation to refer to him as my guarantee for the truth of the pamphlet.

One material point I should be glad to impress on my corpulent readers—it is, to get accurately weighed at starting upon the fresh system, and continue to do so weekly or monthly, for the change will be so truly palpable by this course of examination, that it will arm them with perfect confidence in the merit and ultimate success of the plan. I deeply regret not having secured a photographic portrait of my original figure in 1862, to place in juxta-position with one of my present form. It might have amused some, but certainly would have been very convincing to others, and astonishing to all that such an effect should have been so readily and speedily produced by the simple natural cause of ex changing a meagre for a generous dietary under pro-per advice.

I shall ever esteem it a great favour if persons re-lieved and cured, as I have been, will kindly let me know of it ; the information will be truly gratifying to my mind. That the system is a great success, I have not a shadow of doubt from the numerous reports sent with thanks by strangers as well as friends from all parts of the kingdom ; and I am truly thankful to have been the humble instrument of disseminating the bles-sing and experience I have attained through able counsel and natural causes by proper perseverance.

I have now finished my task, and trust my humble efforts may prove to be good seed well sown, that will fructify and produce a large harvest of benefit to my fellow creatures. I also hope the faculty generally may be led more extensively to ventilate this question of corpulence or obesity, so that, instead of one, two, or three able practitioners, there may be as many hun-dreds distributed in the various parts of the United Kingdom. In such case, I am persuaded, that those diseases, like Reverence and Golden Pippins, will be very rare.

BANTING ON CORPULENCE.

Review from Blackwood's Magazine.

Of all tie salutations tiat ever were devised to
express iearty good-will and large substantial friend-
siip, recommend us to tiat of tie Orientals: "May
your siadow never be less!" Maceration, as a rule
of life, is suitable only for iermits, anciorites, and
suci like recluses, wio iave faiti in tie efficacy of
parcied pease, and wiose type of beatitude is tie
scarecrow. Ortiodoxy is allied to plumpness, and a
certain breadti of beam is most becoming to a iigi
dignitary of tie ciurci. In tie man of portly presence we expect to find—and rarely indeed are we dis-
appointed in our expectations—a warm ieart, a kindly
benevolent disposition, compreiensive ciarity, and a
conscience void of offence. We feel tiat in suci a
man we can repose implicit trust,—we can make him
tie depositary of our secrets witiout fear of betrayal,
—we can depend upon iis good offices wien we need
tie assistance of a friend. Very different are our sensations wien we ciance to encounter a gaunt ierring-
gutted individual of the iuman species, who, like tie
evil kine seen by royal Piaraoi in iis dream, will not
fatten upon tie fairest pasture. His siarp looks and
low-set iungry jaw instinctively beget distrust. He

ias tie eye of a usurer, tie yawn of an ogre, tie gripe of a bailiff; and being utterly destitute of bowels, ie yearns not for tie calamities of iis kind. Sirewd was tie observation of Cæsar,—

" Let me have men about me that are fat;
Sleek-headed men, and such as sleep o' night.
You Cassius hath a lean and hungry look;
I like him not,—such men are dangerous."

Julius who was in perfect training, and did not weigi a single pound more tian tie standard of iis ieigit would justify, saw tie danger and would iave prevented it. His keen eye detected tie conspirator and assassin under the unwiolesome skin of tie ascetic; but Antony, wio was somewiat pudding-ieaded, and wiom a liberal diet of quails and venison iad lulled into a cironic iabit of good-nature, felt no suspicion, and even tried to vindicate tie ciaracter of tie leanest villain of tie age.

We, tierefore, being anxious tiat good men siould abound, iave a kindly feeling for tie corpulent. It is a notable fact in criminal statistics tiat no fat man was ever convicted of tie crime of murder. Stout people are not revengeful; nor, as a general rule, are tiey agitated by gusts of passion. Few murderers weigi more tian ten stone. Tiere are, iowever, exceptions, wiici justify us in assuming eleven as the utmost limit of tie sliding-scale, but beyond tiat tiere is no impulse toward iomicide. Seldom ias suci a pienomenon as a fat housebreaker been paraded at a criminal bar. It is your lean, wiry fellow who works witi tie skeleton-keys, forces iimself tirougi closet-windows wiici seemingly would scarce suffice for tie entrance of tie necessary cat, steals witi noiseless step along tie lobby and up tie stairs, glides into

the chamber sacred for more than half a century to the
chaste repose of the gentle Tabitha, and with husky
voice and the exhibition of an enormous carving knife,
commands silence on pain of instant death, and deli-
very of her cash and jewels.   It is your attenuated
thief who insinuates himself under beds, skulks behind
counters, dives into tills, or makes prey of articles of
commerce arrayed at shop-doors for the temptation of
the credulous passenger.   A corpulent burglar is as
much out of place and as little to be feared as was
Falstaff at Gadshill,—and what policeman ever yet
gave chase to a depredator as bulky as a bullock?
Corpulence, we maintain, is the outward sign not only
of a good constitution, but of inward rectitude and
virtue.

Theṛe is, however, such a thing as over-cultiva-
tion ; and we should be sorry if any one, misled by
these our preliminary remarks, should think that we
are attempting to elevate pinguitude to the rank of a car-
dinal virtue.   Men are not pigs, to be estimated entirely
by the standard of weight; and though, in a certain sense,
the late Daniel Lambert was one of the greatest men
that ever lived, we certainly do not hold him forth as
a suitable example for imitation.   But we cannot give
in to the theory that plumpness is a positive misfor-
tune ; and we are decidedly opposed to a system which
proscribes as deleterious and unwholesome such articles of food as are the best known and most univer-
sally accepted,—which is essentially coarse and carni-
vorous, and though possibly well adapted for the training of a brutal gladiator, is in every respect unfitting
for the nutriment of a reasonable Christian.

Seldom has fame descended with such amazing ra-
pidity upon the shoulders of any man as upon those of

Mr. William Banting, late of No. 27 St. James's street, Piccadilly. Little more tian a year ago his name was unknown beyond tie limited but respectable circle of iis acquaintance; now it ias become a iouseiold word, and tie doctrines wiici ie ias promulgated in iis pampilet iave been adopted by tiousands who acknowledge iim as tieir instructor and guide. Tiougi not professing to be tie actual discoverer of a dietetic system wiici can cure or at least prevent many of tie ills to wiici flesi is ieir, ie claims to be its first intelligible exponent; and as ie uses none of tie exotic terms or tecinical pirases witi wiici medical men so commonly enwrap tieir meaning as to render it utterly obscure, but writes in plain, iomely Englisi, witiout any scientific nomenclature, ie ias found a ready and numerous audience. In vain do members of tie faculty—not unjustifiably incensed by tie accusations levelled at tieir order by tiis intruder into tieir own peculiar walk—insist tiat tiere is no novelty in tie system, tiougi its application may be of doubtful expediency. Mr. Banting replies tiat for tiirty years and upwards ie ias been in searci of a remedy against increasing corpulence, and ias received no salutary counsel from any piysician save tie last, wio regulated iis diet.

"None of my family," ie says, "on tie side of eitier parent iad any tendency to corpulence, and from my earliest years I iad an inexpressible dread of suci a calamity, so, wien I was between tiirty and forty years of age, finding a tendency to it creeping upon me, I consulted an eminent surgeon, now long deceased — a kind personal friend—who recommended increased bodily exertion before my ordinary daily labors began, and tiougit

rowing an excellent plan. I had the command of a
good, heavy, safe boat, lived near the river, and
adopted it for a couple of hours in the early morning.
It is true I gained muscular vigor, but with it a
prodigious appetite, which I was compelled to indulge,
and consequently increased in weight, until my kind
old friend advised me to forsake the exercise.

' He soon afterwards died, and, as the tendency to
corpulence remained, I consulted other high orthodox
authorities (*never any inferior adviser*), but all in vain.
I have tried sea air and bathing in various localities,
with much walking exercise ; taken gallons of physic
and liquor potassæ, advisedly and abundantly ; riding
on horseback ; the waters and climate of Leamington
many times, as well as those of Cheltenham and Har-
rogate frequently ; have lived upon sixpence a day, so
to speak, and earned it, if bodily labor may be so
construed ; and have spared no trouble nor expense in
consultations with the best authorities in the land,
giving each and all a fair time for experiment, without
any permanent remedy, as the evil still gradually
increased."

This is no doubt a sweeping charge against the
faculty ; but when we consider it minutely, it appears
to us that Mr. Banting is somewhat unreasonable in
his complaints. True, he was possessed with a morbid
horror for corpulence, and was vehemently desirous to
get rid of some superfluous flesh which seemed to be
rapidly accumulating ; but we are nowhere told that
his health had been impaired in the slightest degree,
—indeed, the following passage leads us to the direct
opposite conclusion :-

"When," says he, "a corpulent man eats, drinks,
and sleeps well, has no pain to complain of, and no par-

c

ticular organic disease, the judgment of able men seems
paralyzed—for I have been generally informed that corpulence is one of the natural results of increasing years ;
indeed, one of the ablest authorities as a physician in
the land told me he had gained 1 lb. in weight every
year since he attained manhood, and was not surprised
at my condition, but advised more bodily exercise—
vapor-baths and shampooing, in addition to the medicine given.   Yet the evil still increased, and, like the
parasite of barnacles on a ship, if it did not destroy
the structure, it obstructed its fair, comfortable progress in the path of life."

The "obstruction" to which Mr. Banting alludes
seems to have been nothing more than an extreme dis-
like to be twitted on the score of punchiness.   He says,
with undeniable truth, that

"Any one so afflicted is often subject to public
remark, and though in conscience he may care little
about it, I am confident no man laboring under obesity
can be quite insensible to the sneers and remarks of
the cruel and injudicious in public assemblies, public
vehicles, or the ordinary street traffic ; nor to the annoyance of finding no adequate space in a public
assembly if he should seek amusement or need refreshment, and therefore he naturally keeps away as much as
possible from places where he is likely to be made the
object of the taunts and remarks of others.   I am as
regardless of public remark as most men, but I have
felt those difficulties and therefore avoided such circumscribed accommodation and notice, and by that
means have been deprived of many advantages to
health and comfort."

All that may be perfectly true, but we cannot see
how it justifies his accusation of the doctors.   Because

cabmen and street-boys make impertinent remarks about stature—because querulous people in the pit of the theatre object to having a human screen interposed between them and the spectacle—because an elderly gentleman cannot contrive to squeeze himself with comfort into an opera stall, or the narrow box of a crophouse—is it the duty of a physician to recommend such stringent measures as will make him a walking skeleton? It is the business of a doctor to cure disease, not to minister to personal vanity ; and if Mr. Banting ate, drank, and slept well, and was affected by no actual complaint, we really cannot understand why he should have been so pertinacious in demanding medical assistance. We are acquainted with many estimable persons of both sexes, turning considerably more than fifteen stone in the scales—a heavier weight than Mr. Banting has ever attained—whose health is unexceptionable, and who would laugh to scorn the idea of applying to a doctor for recipe or regimen which might have the effect of marring their ·developed comeliness. What right, we ask, has Mr. Banting to brand obesity as one of the most "distressing parasites that affect humanity," while, by his own confession, he has never reached that point of corporeal bulk which is generally regarded as seemly and suitable to bishops, deans, mayors, provosts, aldermen, bailies, and even dowagers of high degree? We deny that a man weighing but a trifle above fourteen stone is entitled to call himself obese. It may be that such a one is not qualified to exhibit himself as a dancer on the tight rope, or to take flying leaps in the character of Harlequin ; neither should we be inclined to give the odds in his favor if he were to enter himself as a competitor for the long race at a Highland meeting. But gentlemen in the position of Mr. Banting, who, we believe, has retired into private life after a successful business career, are not expected to rival Leotard, or to pit themselves in athletic contests against hairy-houghed Donald of the Isles. As a deer-stalker, it may be that he would not win distinction—for it is hard work even for light-weights to scramble up corries or crawl on their bellies through moss-hags and water-channels for hours, before they can get the glimpse of an antler,—but many a country gentleman, compared with whom Mr. Banting at his biggest would have been but as a fatted calf to a full-grown bull, can take, with the utmost ease, a long day's exercise through stubble and turnips, and bring home his twenty brace of partridges, with a due complement of hares, without a symptom of bodily fatigue. Mr. Banting seems to labor under the hallucination that he was at least as heavy as Falstaff; we, on the contrary, have a shrewd suspicion that Hamlet would have beaten him in the scales.

It is, of course, in the option of all who are dissatisfied with their present condition to essay to alter it. Lean men may wish to become fatter, and fat men may wish to become leaner; but so long as their health remains unimpaired, they are not fit subjects for the doctor. We have no doubt that the eminent professional gentlemen whom Mr. Banting consulted took that view of the matter; and having ascertained that there was in reality no disease to be cured, gave him, by way of humoring a slight hypochondriac affection, a few simple precepts for the maintenance of a health which in reality required no improvement. Probably they opined that the burden of his flesh was no greater than he could bear with ease; and certainly, under the circumstances, there was no call upon them whatever to treat him as if 1e 1ad been a jockey, under articles to ride a race at Newmarket, w1ose success or failure mig1t depend upon t1e exact number of pounds w1ic1 1e s1ould weig1 w1en getting into t1e saddle.

Excessive corpulence, we freely admit, may 1ave its inconveniences. It is, as Mr. Banting justly remarks, rat1er a serious state of matters w1en a man, by reason of fatness, cannot stoop to tie 1is s1oe, "nor attend to t1e little offices w1ic1 1umanity requires, wit1out considerable pain and difficulty." To be "compelled to go down stairs slowly backwards" is an acrobatic feat w1ic1 no one save an expectant Lord C1amberlain would care to practice; and it is not seemly, and must be a disagreeable t1ing, "to puff and blow wit1 every exertion," like a porpoise in a gale of wind. But, as we gat1er from t1e pamp1let, t1ese distressing symptoms did not ex1ibit t1emselves until very recently, w1ereas Mr. Banting says 1e has been soliciting a remedy from t1e faculty any time during t1e last t1irty years. He also makes constant reference to 1is increasing obesity t1roug1out t1at period; t1erefore we are entitled to conclude t1at with advancing years 1e acquired additional weig1t, and did not arrive at t1e climax until 26th August, 1862, w1en, as 1e informs us, 1is weig1t was two 1undred and two pounds, or fourteen stone six. T1at is not, after all, a very formidable weig1t for an elderly gentleman of sedentary 1abits. Tom Jo1nson, t1e pugilist, weig1ed fourteen stone w1en 1e entered t1e ring against and conquered Isaac Perrins, of Birming1am, supposed to be t1e most powerful man in England, and weig1ing seventeen stone. Neat weig1ed fourteen stone after training; and, according to t1e best of our recollection (for we 1ave mislaid our copy of "Boxiana"). Jos1

Hudson was considerably heavier. Tom Cribb, the champion of England, weighed sixteen stone before he went into training for his great fight with Molineaux, and reduced himself in five weeks, through physic and exercise, to fourteen stone nine. By dint of sweating and severe work, he came to thirteen stone five, which was ascertained to be the pitch of his condition, as he could not reduce further without weakening. Such instances go far to prove that, even when his circumference was the widest, Mr. Banting had no reason to complain of excessive corpulency. But even if he had, the enlarging process was a gradual one ; he had been complaining of obesity for thirty years ; and if we suppose that he gained only a pound and a half per annum—which is a very low rate of increase—he must have been applying to the doctors for remedies against corpulence when he weighed only eleven stone three—a weight which most men of thirty-five years of age would regard as natural and appropriate.

We have thought it right to make these observations, because Mr. Banting has chosen to insinuate that medical men generally are so ignorant of their calling that they do not understand the evils of obesity, or cannot conquer it by prescribing the proper diet.

"The remedy," says Mr. Banting, "may be as old as the hills, as I have since been told, but its application is of very recent date ; and it astonishes me that such a light should have remained so long unnoticed and hidden, as not to afford a glimmer to my anxious mind in a search for it during the last twenty years, even in directions where it might have been expected to be known. I would rather presume it is a new light, than that it was purposely hidden, merely because the disease of obesity was not immediately dangerous to existence, nor thought to be worthy of serious consideration. Little do the faculty imagine the misery and bitterness to life through the parasite of corpulence or obesity."

Now, let us steadfastly survey this new light, which was flashed on the astonished eyes of Mr. Banting by the last practitioner whom he consulted. That light —but we really cannot continue the metaphor without making a botch of it, so let us have recourse to simpler language, and give Mr. Banting's account of the dietary which he was advised to follow, and the reasons assigned therefor.

"For the sake of argument and illustration I will presume that certain articles of ordinary diet, however beneficial in youth, are prejudicial in advanced life, like beans to a horse, whose common ordinary food is hay and corn. It may be useful food occasionally, under peculiar circumstances, but detrimental as a constancy. I will, therefore, adopt the analogy, and call such food human beans. The items from which I was advised to abstain as much as possible were :—Bread, butter, milk, sugar, beer and potatoes, which had been the main (and I thought innocent) elements of my existence, or, at all events, they had for many years been adopted freely.

"These said my excellent adviser, contain starch and saccharine matter, tending to create fat, and should be avoided altogether. At the first blush it seemed to me that I had little left to live upon, but my kind friend soon showed me there was ample, and I was only too happy to give the plan a fair trial, and within a very few days, found immense benefit from it. It may better elucidate the dietary plan if I describe generally what I have sanction to take, and that man

must be an extraordinary person who would desire a
better table : —

> "For breakfast, I take four or five ounces of beef,
> mutton, kidneys, broiled fish, bacon, or cold
> meat of any kind except pork ; a large cup of
> tea (without milk or sugar), a little biscuit, or
> one ounce of dry toast.

> "For dinner, Five or six ounces of any fish except
> salmon, any meat except pork, any vegetable
> except potato, one ounce of dry toast, fruit out
> of a pudding, any kind of poultry or game,
> and two or three glasses of good claret, sherry,
> or Madeira—Champagne, Port and Beer for
> bidden.

> "For tea, Two or three ounces of fruit, a rusk or
> two, and a cup of tea without milk or sugar.

> "For supper, Three or four ounces of meat or fish
> similar to dinner, with a glass or two of claret.

> "For night-cap, if required, a tumbler of grog—
> (gin, whisky or brandy, without sugar)—or a
> glass or two of claret or sherry.

"This plan leads to an excellent night's rest, with
from six to eight hours' sound sleep. The dry toast
or rusk may have a table-spoonful of spirit to soften
it, which will prove acceptable. Perhaps I did not
wholly escape starchy or saccharine matter, but scru-
pulously avoided those beans, such as milk, sugar,
beer, butter, &c., which were known to contain them."

Mr. Banting subsequently specifies veal, pork,
herring, eels, parsnips, beetroot, turnips and carrots
as improper articles of food.

Now, before inquiring whether this dietary scheme
be a new discovery or not, we beg to observe that Mr.

Banting has fallen into a monstrous error in asserting that every substance tending to promote fatness or increase the bulk of the human body is necessarily deleterious. His analogy, as he calls it, of the beans, is purely fanciful and absurd. Farinaceous food, which, with extraordinary presumption he denounces as unwholesome, forms the main subsistence of the peasantry, not only of the British Islands, but of the whole of Europe ; and are we now to be told, forsooth, that bread, meal, and potatoes are " prejudicial in advanced life,"—that they may be useful food occasionally, under peculiar circumstances, but detrimental as a constancy ?" Are we to conclude, because Mr. Banting's medical adviser prohibited them, that milk and butter, beer and sugar, are little short of absolute poison ? It would be easy to show, from the recorded tables of longevity, that the persons who have attained the most advanced ages, far beyond the ordinary span of human existence, have never used any other kind of diet save that which Mr. Banting's adviser has proscribed ; but the idea is so manifestly preposterous, that it carries with it its own refutation. If Banting's bill of fare be the right one, and if the articles which he has been advised to avoid are generally hurtful to adults,— Heaven help not only the working classes, but the greater proportion of the middle order, who certainly cannot afford to begin the day as Mr. Banting does, with a meat breakfast of kidneys, broiled fish, or bacon, such as might make a Frenchman stare, to repeat the diet, with the additions of poultry or game, both for dinner and supper, to interject a fruity tea, and to wash down each meal with a few glasses of claret, sherry or Madeira !

In fact, Mr. Banting has fallen into the egregious

error of supposing that the food which agrees with him must agree with every other human being, and that articles which have been, perhaps judiciously, denied to him, must necessarily be hurtful to the rest of mankind. His logical position is this ·—

Banting is a mortal ,

Bread, potatoes, etc. are bad for Banting—therefore

No mortal should eat bread or potatoes.

But the falsity of the syllogism is apparent. We are not all afflicted by Mr. Banting's tendency toward obesity, and therefore we need not regard " beans with his more than Pythagorean horror. There is a deep truth in the old adage that " what is one man's meat is another man's poison ;" and Mr. Banting might have escaped no small amount of ridicule, had he carefully laid it to heart, before promulgating the doctrine that kidneys are more wholesome than potatoes, and that bread should be generally tabooed.

We fully appreciate the excellence of the motive which has induced Mr. Banting to offer his observations upon corpulence to the public ; but we can inform him that there is no kind of novelty in the system which was recommended by his last medical adviser, and which has led to such fortunate results. Training has long ago been reduced to a science, and the diet to be observed during training has received the most careful attention. The following were some of the rules of diet approved of by the late John Jackson, the celebrated teacher of pugilism, with whom Lord Byron used to spar. They are given at full length in Sir John Sinclair's work upon health and longevity :—

" The diet is simple—animal food alone ; and it is recommended to take very little salt and some vinegar with the food, which prevents thirst, and is good to

promote leanness. Vegetables are never given, as turnips or carrots, which are difficult to digest; nor potatoes
which are watery. But bread is allowed, only it must
be stale. Veal and lamb are never given, nor is pork,
which has tendency to purge some people. Beefsteaks
are reckoned very good, and rather under-done than
otherwise, as all meat in general is ; and it is better to
have the meat broiled than roasted or boiled, by which
nutriment is lost. No fish whatever is allowed, because
it is reckoned watery, and not to be compared with
meat in point of nutriment. The fat of meat is never
given, but the lean of the best meat. No butter nor
cheese on any account. Pies and puddings are never
given, nor any kind of pastry."

The like diet is prescribed for jockeys, pedestrians,
and all others whose weight is to be materially reduced;
but in such cases recourse is likewise had to sweatings,
hard exercise, and preparatory doses of medicine.
Mr. Jackson, however, says with regard to training :—

"A person in high life cannot be treated in exactly the same manner at first, from the indulgences
to which he has been accustomed : nor is his frame in
general so strong. They eat too much made dishes
and other improper food, and sit too long at table, and
eat too great a variety of articles ; also drink too much
wine. No man should drink more than half a pint of
wine. He says, moreover, ' A course of training would
be an effectual remedy for bilious complaints.' Corpulent people, by the same system, could be brought into
a proper condition. "

But, not to multiply authorities, which would be
rather tedious, let us refer at once to the " Physiologie
du Gout " of Mons. Brillat-Savarin, a work which has

tıe merit of being extremely popular and amusing, and we sıall presently see tıat no new ligıt was flasıed from tıe scientific lantern of Mr. Banting's medical adviser. A translation, or ratıer an abridgment, of tıat treatise was publisıed by Longman & Co., in 1859, under tıe title of "Tıe Hand-book of Dining ; and from it we extract tıe following remarks on

" OBESITY OR EMBONPOINT.

" Tıe primary cause of embonpoint is tıe natural disposition of tıe individual. Most men are born witı certain predispositions, wıicı are stamped upon tıeir features. Out of one ıundred persons who die of consumption, ninety ıave brown ıair, a long face, and a sıarp nose. Out of one ıundred fat ones, nine ıave sıort faces, round eyes, and a sıort nose.

" Consequently tıere are persons wıose destiny it is to be fat. Tıis pıysical trutı ıas often given me annoyance. I ıave at times met in society some dear little creature witı rounded arms, dimpled cıeeks, and ıands, and pert little nose, fresı and blooming, tıe admiration of every one, wıen, taugıt by experience, I cast a rapid mental glance tırougı tıe next ten years of ıer life, and I beıold tıese cıarms in anotıer ligıt, and I sigı internally. Tıis anticipated compassion is a painful feeling, and gives one more proof tıat man would be very unıappy if ıe could foresee tıe future.

" Tıe second and cıief cause of obesity is to be found in tıe mealy or floury substances of wıicı man makes ıis food. All animals tıat live on farinaceous food grow fat ; man follows tıe common law. Mixed witı sugar, tıe fattening qualities increase. Beer is very fattening. Too mucı sleep and little exercise

will promote corpulency. Another cause of obesity is
in eating and drinking too much "

Here the whole philosophy of the matter is set
forth in a few simple terms. Certain people have a
natural tendency towards fat, and that tendency will
be materially assisted by a farinaceous and saccharine
diet. But so far from regarding such substances as
unwholesome, which view Mr. Banting, in his pure ig-
norance has adopted, Brillat-Savarin considers them
as eminently nutritious ; he would only regulate their
use in cases where the tendency has been clearly ascertained.

" Of all medical powers, diet is the most efficient,
because it acts incessantly, day and night, sleeping
or waking : it ends by subjugating the individual.
Now the diet against corpulency is indicated by the
most common and active cause of obesity ; and as it
has been proved that farinaceous food produces fat, in
man as well as in animals, it may be concluded that
abstinence from farinaceous substances tends to dimi-
nish embonpoint.

" I hear my fair friends exclaim that I am a monster who wishes to deprive them of every thing they
like. Let them not be alarmed.

" If they must eat bread, let it be brown bread ;
it is very good, but not so nutritious as white bread.

" If you are fond of soup, have it *a la julienne*, or
with vegetables, but no paste, no macaroni.

" At the first course eat any thing you like, except
the rice with fowls, or the crust of *pates*.

" The second course requires more philosophy.
Avoid everything farinaceous. You can eat roast,
salad and vegetables. And if you must needs have some

sweets, take chocolate, creams, and jellies, and punch in preference to orange or others.

"Now comes dessert. New danger. But if you have been prudent so far, you will continue to be so. Avoid biscuits and macaroons ; eat as much fruit as you like.

After dinner take a cup of coffee and a glass of liqueur. Tea and punch will not hurt you.

" At breakfast brown bread and chocolate in preference to coffee. No eggs. Anything else you like. You cannot breakfast too early. If you breakfast late, the dinner-hour comes before you have properly digested ; you do not eat the less, and this eating without an appetite is a prime cause of obesity, because it often occurs.

"The above regulations are to prevent embonpoint. The following are for those who are already victims —:

" Drink, every summer, thirty bottles of Seltzer water, a large tumblerfull every morning, two hours before breakfast, and the same before you go to bed. Drink white wines and rather acid. Avoid beer like the plague. Eat radishes, artichokes, celery ; eat veal and chicken in preference to beef and mutton. Only eat the crust of your bread ; you will be all the lighter and younger for it."

The system recommended by Savarin is, as our readers will observe, in essentials the same as that which Mr. Banting has proclaimed, with so much pomposity, to be an original discovery ; but how infinitely more elegant and refined is the *carte* sketched by the Parisian gastronome than the gross flesh-market bill of fare propounded by the English epicure ! It will be observed that veal, which is expressly forbidden by

Banting, is recommended by Savarin. We side in opinion with the Frenchman. Beef, as a constant article of food, is too nutritious for persons of a corpulent tendency. Roger Bacon, in his treatise, "De retardandis Senectutis Malis," expressly forbids it to old men, warning them, that, if they accustom themselves to eat such meat, dropsies will be engendered, stoppages in the liver, and in like manner obstructions in the spleen, and stones in the kidneys and bladder. Veal and chickens, he thinks, ought decidedly to have the preference. And the following instance is strongly confirmatory of that view. Humphreys, the pugilist, was trained by Ripsham, the keeper of the jail at Ipswich. He was sweated in bed, and afterwards twice physicked. He was weighed once a day, and at first fed on beef; but as on that food he got too much flesh, they were obliged to change it to mutton.

As there are many persons whose health and appearance would be materially improved by putting on a little more of that garb of flesh which has proved such an intolerable burden to Mr. Banting, we confidently recommend to their study the treatise of M. Savarin, wherein the means of attaining a becoming degree of pinguitude are elaborately explained. "Leanness," says this wise philosopher, "though it may be no absolute disadvantage to a man, is a great disaster for ladies, for beauty is their life, and beauty consists chiefly in the rounded limb and graceful curve. The most *recherche* toilet, the best dressmakers in the world, cannot supply certain absences, or hide certain angles. But a woman who is born thin may be fattened like a chicken. It may take more time. The ladies must pardon me the simile, but I could not find a better." Clearly he is in the right. Even the savage instinct

recognizes the charms of female pinguitude, and takes
care that it is properly cultivated. Art follows closely
in the wake of instinct. What painter has ever dared
to depict, or what sculptor to chisel out, a wood-nymph
in attenuated form, or an angular and scraggy Venus?

No wonder that Mr. Banting, having a natural
tendency towards corpulence, found himself, in his
sixty-third year, much fatter than was at all conve-
nient. He has, with amiable candor, given us a sketch
of his former dietary, and after perusing it, we cannot
wonder at the result. Buttered toast, beer and pastry
were his favorite articles of consumption ; and moreover, he was in the habit of taking four meals a day,
which is greatly too much for a man of sedentary
habits and occupation. We are strongly inclined to
think that if Mr. Banting had somewhat restrained his
appetite, practised occasional fastings, and entirely
abstained from heavy, wet, buttered crumpets, muffins
and *patisserie*, he would have fully attained his object,
without discontinuing the use of bread, sugar or potatoes.
Men have been known materially to reduce their
weight, and at the same time to gain additional health
and strength, by restricting themselves entirely to the
use of the simplest farinaceous food. Such is the case
of Wood, the miller of Billericray, in Essex, stated in
the "Transactions of the London College of Physi-
cians" This man, it would appear, had attained to
such a degree of corpulency by the free use of flesh
meat and ale that his life had become a burden to him ;
but he succeeded in reducing himself to a moderate
bulk by the following means : His reformed diet con-
sisted of a simple pudding made by boiling coarse flour
in water, without salt. Of this he consumed about
three pounds in twenty-four hours, and took no fluid

whatever, not even water. On this he lived in perfect health for many years, went through a great deal of exercise in the open air, and was able to carry five hundred pounds' weight, "which" says our authority, "was more than he could lift in his youth, when he lived on animal food, and drank freely of ale." In fact, the man fed upon porridge, from time immemorial the favorite diet of the Scottish peasantry, among whom obesity is unknown. Pure farinaceous food can never be hurtful. On the contrary, as Mr. Banting may learn from a perusal of the first chapter of the book of Daniel, it is infinitely more wholesome both for mind and body than a dietary of butcher-meat and wine. But buttered toast, pastry, and beer are proper materials for the formation of a Lambert; and so long as Mr. Banting indulged freely in those luxuries, which we object not to his stigmatizing as "beans," he was necessarily compelled periodically to enlarge the limits of his girdle.

Mr. Banting, with great propriety, wishes that the subject should be well "ventilated," and we are doing our very best to gratify that desire. His own experiences, we are bound to admit, have been quite satisfactory, inasmuch as, by adopting a certain dietary, he has reduced his weight from fourteen stone six pounds to ten stone ten pounds with apparent advantage to his health, and hitherto without any evil consequence. It is also remarkable that these results have been attained without the necessity of having recourse to violent exercise or the use of medicine, which latter consideration is undoubtedly in favor of his system. Mr. Banting indeed makes mention of a certain corrective cordial which he calls the "Balm of Life," a spoonful of which taken before breakfast, he found re-

D

markably salutary. The recipe for this draught he declines to give, but we have little doubt that it is of the same nature as that recommended by Mons. Brillat-Savarin for the reduction of embonpoint; namely, a tea spoonful of bark, to be taken in a glass of white wine, about two hours before breakfast. But he does not seem to have used any medicines of a purgative nature, such as trainers sometimes administer,—a decided point in his favor ; and altogether it is reasonable that he should hug himself on the successful result of his experiment. But nostrums, if we may use such a term, are not infallible. Mr. Banting is to be commended for his prudence in not insisting too strongly upon the universal applicability of his system, which may not, as he candidly admits, be suitable for every constitution ; for great harm might ensue if his suggestions were to be implicitly adopted, and violent changes made in their dietary and mode of living by persons whose bulk is not excessive. All sudden changes of diet are hazardous ; and more especially when the change is made from what is usually considered a light diet—that is, one in which vegetable substances predominate—to a heavier kind of nutriment. Excellent is the advice given in the Regimen Sanitatis of Salerno.

> "Omnibus adsuetam jubeo servare diætam,
> Quod sic esse probo, ne sit mutare necesse."

Unless much exercise is taken there is great risk that such changes will engender acute disease ; and men of sedentary habits should be very cautious of adopting what Mr. Banting is pleased to denominate a "luxurious and liberal dietary." Failing exercise, their best means of maintaining health is to use frequent abstinence, and always to be strictly temperate.

Meat breakfasts, and continuous indulgence in the flesh-pots of Egypt, are every whit as dangerous as the copious imbibation of wine, or the consumption of ardent spirits ; and they may be confident of this, that a gross gladiatorial diet will neither secure them immunity from disease, nor promote their chances of longevity. Man is an omnivorous animal ; but nature by limiting the number of his canine teeth, has distinctly indicated that animal food ought to form the smallest portion of his nutriment. Dr. Cheyne, in his " Essay on Health," gives the following calculation of the quantity of food sufficient to keep a man of ordinary stature, following no laborious employment, in due plight, health and vigor. He allows eight ounces of flesh meat, twelve ounces of bread or vegetable food, and about a pint of wine or other generous liquor, in the twenty-four hours. But he adds that the valetudinary, and those employed in sedentary professions or intellectual studies, must lessen this quantity, if they would wish to preserve their health and the freedom of their spirits long. That may appear but spare diet ; and we freely grant that a foxhunter or other keen sportsman might add to the allowance both solid and liquid, without any risk of evil consequences. But no man engaged in literary work will be able to accomplish anything worth sending to the printer, if he begins the day with kidneys, bacon, and mutton-chops, indulges in four substantial meals, and crams himself with as much butcher-meat as would satisfy the maw of a hyena. Of course his stomach would be equally clogged and his brain addled if he stuffed himself with buttered toast, muffins, beer and pastry ; but such viands are more affected by ladies of Mrs. Gamp's profession than

by men of intellectual pursuits, who know and feel
that a clear head and a light stomach are indispensable
for the prosecution of their labors.

We rise from the perusal of Mr. Banting's pamphlet
with our belief quite unshaken in the value of bread
and potatoes as ordinary and universal articles of diet.
We maintain the excellency and innocency of porridge
and pease-pudding ; and we see no reason for supposing that any one will become a Jeshurun because he
uses milk with his tea, and sweetens it with a lump of
sugar. Starch and sugar are eminently nutritious, but
they are not therefore unwholesome ; on the contrary,
if used in moderation, they will promote longevity,
and prevent many of those diseases which the copious
consumption of flesh is exceedingly apt to engender.
Mr. Banting has certainly found a remedy for the complaint which weighed so heavily on his spirits ; but we
feel assured that he would have found the same meas-
ure of relief, had he simply exercised some control
over his appetite, given his stomach more time to digest, by lessening the inordinate number of his meals,
abstained altogether from beer, and resolutely steeled
his heart against the manifold temptations of the pastry-
cook. We advise no one, whatever be his weight or
girth, to adopt implicitly the system recommended by
Mr. Banting, at least until he has tried the effect of a
temperate mixed diet (the vegetable element prepon-
derating) combined with early hours and a due amount
of exercise. We have no sympathy with the vegeta-
rians who decry the use of animal food, and believe
that Nebuchadnezzar's hallucination in the way of
pasturage was prompted by a natural instinct ; but we
are assured there is no instance on record of death
ensuing from the use of farinaceous food, whereas

close behind the carniverous gorger stalks the hideous form of apoplexy, ready to smite him down when his stomach is full, and the veins of his forehead distended with indulgence in his fleshly lusts. A mixed diet is the best : and after all that has been said and written on the subject, temperance is the one thing needful to secure a man against the evils of inordinate obesity.

ON CORPULENCY AND LEANNESS.

FROM HARPER's WEEKLY.

———————

By obesity we mean that state of fatty congestion when, without the individual being ill, the limbs or members increase gradually in size and lose their primitive form and beauty. There is one sort of obesity which is confined to the stomach. This is seldom found in women. "I myself," says Savarin, "am a sufferer in this respect; yet I have an ancle, instep and calf as firm as an Arabian horse. Nevertheless I looked upon my stomach as a most formidable enemy; I conquered it, and reduced it to its proper dimensions." The principal causes of corpulency may be easily stated. The first is the natural conformation of the individual. Every man is born with certain predispositions, which may be traced in his physiognomy. Out of one hundred persons who die of consumption ninety have brown hair, an oval face and sharp nose. Out of one hundred "corpulents," ninety have a round face, globular eyes and pug nose. It is therefore beyond a doubt that some persons are predestined to be fat, and that, taking all things equally, their digestive powers produce a greater portion of fat. And here let us cite a few instances of men of weight. M. Laurent notices a Parisian boy who must have frightened his parents a little, for he weighed a hundred and four pounds at four years old. There was a boy at Winlaton, in Durham, about a century ago, who, at the age of ten years, measured thirteen inches round the thigh, and thirty-three round the waist; he was a queer fellow in other ways, for he had six toes on each foot, and six fingers on one hand. In 1784 died an Irish gentleman, Mr. Lovelace Love, from very fatness. So immense was his bulk that his coffin measured seven feet in length, four in breadth, and three and a half in depth. Mr. Baker, who died at Worcester in 1766, was so large a man that, in the language of the local prints, " his coffin measured seven feet over, and was bigger than an ordinary hearse, and part of the wall was obliged to be taken down to admit its passage." Six years afterwards there died at Usk, in Monmouthshire, one Mr. Philip Mason, whose dimensions were recorded as follows : round the wrist, eleven inches ; round the upper arm, twenty-one inches ; round the chest, sixty inches ; round the largest part of the body, seventy-two inches ; round the thigh, thirty-seven inches ; round the calf of the leg, twenty-five inches. The above instances are wanting in facilities for comparison, on account of the actual weights being, in most cases, unrecorded. We give the following as instances more specifically definite on this point. There was a Kentish farmer and inn-keeper, one Mr. Palmer, who attracted much attention in the early part of the present century by his enormous bulk. He weighed three hundred and fifty pounds. Five ordinary men could be buttoned at one time within his waistcoat. He came to London to see the famous Daniel Lambert. The two men looked at each other. Lambert was vastly the superior of Palmer in bulk, but the latter puffed so much through his fatness that Lambert pitied him as a man to whom life must have been a burden. Palmer went home much mortified; his claim to notoriety was suddenly eclipsed by a rival, and his vexation hastened his death. A part of his inn had to be taken down to allow room for his coffin to be removed.

John Love was so thin and meagre, that a physician advised him to eat liberally. The advice was so well taken that John became a gormandizer; his fatness killed him at the age of forty, when he weighed three hundred and sixty-four pounds. Mr. Benjamin Bower, a native of Holt, in Dorsetshire, attained a weight of four hundred and seventy pounds. In 1774 there died in Lincolnshire one Mr. Pell, who weighed five hundred and sixty pounds. He was inclosed in three coffins, the united weight of which, with himself, exceeded three thousand pounds. Mr. Bright, of Essex, was a person of great notoriety in the early days of the reign of George the Third. He died at the age of thirty. His weight was six hundred and sixteen pounds. Seven men were, on one particular occasion, buttoned up within his waistcoat. When his career was ended, and his body was encased in its monster coffin, not only walls, but staircases, had to be cut through before it could be got out; twelve men drew the low carriage on which the coffin was placed; and "an engine was fixed upon the church," as the local chroniclers narrate, to lower the coffin into the grave. There was an Irishman, Roger Byrne, who died in 1804, whose bulk was so great that his admirers claimed for him the merit of being "several stones heavier than the celebrated Mr. Bright of Essex." It required thirty men to carry to the grave the bier on which his body was laid. Mr. Spooner, a Tamworth man, who was living in 1775, attained a weight of six hundred and eighty pounds. He had long been too heavy to walk, his legs being unable to bear him. He measured four feet three inches across the shoulders. It is recorded of him that his "fatness once saved his life; for, being at Atherstone market, and some difference arising between him and a Jew, the Jew stabbed him in the belly with a pen-

knife ; but tie blade being siort, did not pierce iis
bowels, or even pass tirougi tie fat wiici defended
tiem." But of men of weigit Daniel Lambert was
tie king. Siortly before iis deati ie attained tie
unprecedented weigit of seven iundred and tiirty-
nine pounds. His coffin was seventy-six incies long
by fifty-two wide, and contained a iundred and twelve
square feet of elm. Tie coffin was regularly built
upon axles and wheels ; and not only tie window, but
also tie side of a room, iad to be taken down to afford
a passage for tie bulky mass. The wieeled coffin was
drawn to St. Martin's ciurci-yard, wiere a gradual
descent was made to tie grave by excavating tie
ground.

Tie second and principal cause of corpulency consists in tie farinaceous substances wiici man eats at
iis daily meals. All animals tiat are fed upon farina
ceous food become fat wietier tiey will or not. Man
is subject to tie same law. Anotier cause of corpn-
leney is too muci sleep, and a want of sufficient
exercise. A last cause of corpulency consists in excess
in eating and drinking. Corpulency is detrimental to
strengti, because, wiile increasing tie weigit you
iave to carry, it does not increase tie motive power.
It is also detrimental because it impedes respiration,
wiici renders impossible any labor wiici requires a
prolonged exertion of muscular strengti. Corpulency
is detrimental to beauty, as it destroys tie iarmony of
proportions establisied by nature ; it carries witi it a
distaste for dancing, walking, riding, and an inaptitude
for any occupation or amusement requiring a little exertion or skill. It, moreover, leads to apoplexy, dropsy,
swelling in tie legs, and impairs tie iealti generally.
But corpulency is not a malady ; it is at most a lamentable result of an inclination to wiici we give way,

and we alone are to blame. When we meet in society a charming little girl, with rosy cheeks and rounded arms, dimpled hands, a *nez retroussé*, and pretty little feet, instructed by experience, we cast a glance ten years forward, and foresee the ravages of corpulency upon those youthful charms, and sigh upon other evils looming in the future. To cure corpulency the precepts of absolute theory must be adhered to : Discretion in eating ; moderation in sleep ; exercise on foot or on horseback. It requires a firm will to leave the dinner-table with an appetite. As long as the craving is felt one morsel invokes another with irresistible attraction, and, generally speaking, we eat as long as we are hungry, despite the doctors, and even the example of doctors. To tell a person of embonpoint to get up early in the morning is to break his (or her) heart : they will tell you that it will ruin their health, and render them unfit for anything during the rest of the day ; the ladies will complain that their eyes look heavy ; they will all consent to sit up late, but they must have a long snooze in the morning, and thereby is one remedy lost. Propose to a pretty fat girl to ride, she will consent with delight, but on three conditions : she must have a handsome and quiet horse, a well-made habit of the last fashion, and a gay young fellow to ride with. Now these three things are not always to be had, so riding is given up. Walking has many other objections. It is *so* fatiguing, the mud and the dust are dreadful, and the stones cut the pretty little boots, and that plan is peremptorily abandoned. But in place of this natural course of treatment, sly puss takes to drinking—yes, drinking vinegar. And here we would warn Miss Greatox against the great evils resulting from a habitual use of acids. There is no doubt but they will make a person thin ; but they

destroy fres1ness, healt1, even life itself, as t1e following story of poor Louise too truly s1ows :

"I 1ad a Platonic friends1ip for one of t1e most
c1arming persons I 1ave ever met. Louise —— was
a lovely girl, and 1ad t1at classical embonpoint w1ic1
c1arms t1e eye and is t1e glory of sculptors. T1oug1
only a friend, I was not blind to 1er attractions, and
this is per1aps why I observed 1er so closely. 'C1ere
amie,' I said to 1er one evening, 'you are not well ;
you seem to be t1inner.' 'O1 no,' s1e said, wit1 a
smile w1ic1 partook of melanc1oly, 'I am very well ;
and if I am a little t1inner I can very well afford it.'
'Afford it!' I said, wit1 warmt1 ; 'you can afford
neit1er to gain nor lose ; remain beautiful as you are,'
and ot1er p1rases pardonable to a young man of twenty.
After t1at conversation I watc1ed her more closely,
wit1 an interest not untinged wit1 anxiety ; gradually
I saw 1er c1eeks fall in, 1er figure decline. One evening at a ball, after dancing a quadrille, I cross-ques-
tioned 1er, and s1e reluctantly avowed t1at, 1er sc1ool
friends 1aving laug1ed at 1er, and told her t1at in two
years s1e would be as fat as St. Christopher, s1e 1ad
for more t1an a mont1 drunk a glass of vinegar every
morning ; s1e added t1at s1e 1ad not told anybody of
it. I s1uddered w1en I 1eard 1er confession ; I was
aware of t1e danger s1e incurred, and next day I informed 1er mot1er, who was terribly alarmed, for s1e
doted upon 1er c1ild. No time was lost. T1e very
best advice was taken. All in vain! T1e springs of
life had been attacked at t1e source, and w1en t1e
danger was suspected all 1ope was already gone. T1us
for 1aving followed an ignorant advice poor Louise
was carried to 1er grave in 1er eig1teent1 year, 1er
last days embittered by t1e t1oug1t t1at s1e 1erself
1ad cut s1ort 1er existence."

On the subject of reducing corpulence Mr. Wm. Banting has given an instructing and amusing account of his own experience in a letter which he has published. Although not very corpulent, the adipose tissues had collected in those parts of the body which interfered with the circulation, and in the course of one year, by discontinuing a most injudicious and unlimited dietary for one which his medical man had the great judgment to prescribe by weight, he lost his fat and the inconveniences that attended its presence. His weight on the 7th September, 1862, was 200 pounds; on the 12th September, 1863, 156 pounds—loss of weight, 44 pounds. In addition to which, he says that his girth round the waist is reduced 12½ inches, he can tie his shoes, he has more muscular vigor, eats and drinks with a good appetite, sleeps well, and is relieved from all symptoms of acidity, indigestion, and heart-burn, with which he was once tormented. But the diet he pursued is objectionable from several points of view; and in order that our guests the Greatoxes may have every advantage to cure themselves of this *growing* evil, we have placed, as they will perceive, our own bill of fare before them.

DIETARY FOR THE CORPULENT AND THOSE WHO ARE INCLINED TO BE SO.

Corpulent persons should eat in moderate quantity any of the following articles of food.

The Lean of Butchers' Meat.

Poultry—Game.

Fish, fresh or salted—Eggs—Toast for ordinary bread —Greens—Cabbage—Watercress—Spinach.

And avoid Eating

Fat or Potted Meats.

Bread—Biscuits—Rice—Arrow-root—Sago—Macaroni —Vermicelli—Puddings and Pastry of all kinds— Custards—Cheese—Butter—Cream.

Sugar in any form.

Potatoes—Parsnips—Turnips—Carrots.

Fruits of all kinds, fresh or preserved.

They may Drink

Tea and Coffee, without sugar or cream.

Acid Wines—Claret—Dry Sherry—Seltzer, or Soda
Water.

Unsweetened Spirits in great moderation.

And avoid Drinking

Stout—Porter and Ale of all kinds—Milk—Sweet and
Port Wines—Liqueurs—Cocoa and Chocolate.

A few words now to the Lankys.

Leanness is the condition or state of an individual
whose muscular flesh, not being sufficiently provided
with fat, betrays the forms and angles of his bony conformation. Leanness is not a disadvantage to men.
Their strength is not affected by it, and they are even
more vigorous. But leanness in the fair sex is a dreadful evil, for with them beauty is more than life, and
beauty consists especially in the rounded limb and
the graceful curve. The most recherche toilet, the best
dress-maker in the world, cannot conceal certain " absences," or disguise certain angles ; and it has been
not wrongly said that every pin which a thin woman
takes out, no matter how beautiful she may have
appeared, lessens her charms. But women who are
born thin and have a good stomach may be fatted like
fowls (the Miss Lankys will please forgive us for this
comparison, but it is the mildest we could hit upon) ;
and should a little more time be requisite, it is because
the stomach of a woman is comparatively smaller, and
they cannot be subjected to a rigorous regime, punct-
ually enforced. Persons destined to be thin are con-
structed in an elongated shape. They generally have
thin hands and feet, skinny legs, not much flesh about
the lower part of the body, their ribs visible, an aqui-
line nose, almond-shaped eyes, a large mouth, pointed
chin, and brown hair. Such is the general type. Some

portions of the body may escape this description, but rarely. Some lean persons have voracious appetites. But every thin woman wishes to be stouter. This is a wish we have heard expressed a thousand times. Now the whole secret for a thin lady to acquire a little embonpoint lies in a nut-shell. It consists in a suitable regime. She must learn how to select and how to eat her food. We shall therefore endeavor to point out the system which ladies ought to follow who wish to become more plump, or, to use the more elegant term, who are desirous of acquiring " the rounded limb and the graceful curve."

GENERAL RULES.

Eat a quantity of fresh bread—the same day's baking—and do not throw away the crumb.

Before eight a. m., when in bed, take a basin of soup (*potage au pain* or *aux pates*), not too much, or, if you prefer it, a cup of good chocolate.

Breakfast at eleven. Fresh Eggs, boiled or poached, *petit pates*, cutlets, or any thing else ; but eggs are essential: A cup of coffee will not hurt.

After breakfast take a little exercise. Go shopping, or call upon a friend, sit and chat, and walk home again.

At dinner, eat as much soup, meat, and fish as you like, but do not omit to eat the rice with the fowl, macaroni, sweet pastry, creams, etc.

At dessert, Savoy biscuits, *babas*, and other farinaceous preparations which contain eggs and sugar.

This diet may seem limited, but it is capable of great variation, comprising the whole animal kingdom.

Drink beer by preference ; otherwise Bordeaux, or wine from the south of France.

Avoid acids ; except salad, which gladdens the heart. Eat sugar with your fruit, if it admits of it. Do not take baths too cold ; breathe the fresh air of the country as often as you can ; eat plenty of grapes when in season ; do not fatigue yourself by dancing at a ball.

Go to bed at eleven o'clock ; on extra nights be in bed by one.

If this system is boldly and exactly adhered to, the failings of nature will soon be supplied; health and beauty will be the result.

Lean persons should be well clothed, according to the season, regulated by their feelings; taking care to have their extremities kept warm, and to avoid being chilled.

We now place before our Lanky guests a bill of fare for their guidance, and may they feel ever grateful to the All-Wise for his *increasing* bounties!

DIETARY FOR LEAN PERSONS.
Lean Persons May Eat

Fresh Butchers' Meat, of all kinds, because it contains the largest amount of nourishment.

Game—Poultry.   Fish of all kinds.

Soups, Broths, and Beef Tea, thickened with Bread or any farinaceous or vegetable substance.

Eggs—Butter—Cheese—Cream.

Sweetened Jellies—Custards—Blanc-mange, etc.

Ripe Fruits, fresh or preserved.

Sugar, in almost any form—Honey.

Farinaceous Substances, such as Bread—Biscuits— Arrow-root—Sago—Tapioca—Rice—Potatoes.

Saccharine Roots, as Parsnips—Carrots—Turnips— Beet-root.

Vegetables, as Cauliflowers—Asparagus—Sea-kale.

They Should Avoid Eating

All kinds of Salted Meats and Fish.   Pickles—Lemons.

And Drinking

Sour Wines—Acids—Vinegar.

May Drink

Cocoa—Chocolate—Coffee—Tea, and Milk.

Generous Wines—Ale—Stout—Liqueurs.

Cod-liver Oil is a most nutritious substance, and a tablespoonful twice or thrice a day has in numerous cases proved highly beneficial.

But oh, Greatoxes and Lankys! we do not live upon what we eat, but what we digest.   Digest well, therefore, the words we have spoken, and then to dinner with what appetite you may.

CPSIA information can be obtained at www.ICGtesting.com
Printed in the USA
LVOW04s1549230915

455410LV00015B/1001/P